The 7 Habits for a better sleep

A practical guide to building long-lasting habits

CALLIE MORENO

information contained within this document, including, but not limited to, — errors, omissions, or inaccuracies.

CONTENTS

INTRODUCTION

Anytime we want to build new habits, we jump straight into it, and we find ourselves failing after a couple of weeks. Have you ever wondered why? You can create successful habits when you have a robust structure.

If YOU want to build successful habits, this book provides the tools to build long-lasting habits and shares seven easy habits to improve yours. Through the conscious awareness of these practices, you will benefit not only when sleeping but also experience an improvement in your daily routine. These practices will improve your focus and energy level.

Callie Moreno was born in Ecuador, immigrated to Spain when she was 13. She moved to London and graduated in Medical Bioscience. Callie is an authority because of her passion for self-awareness and psychology studies. Her bad sleeping patterns for many years led her to study conscious habits that would improve her routine. These habits have become part of her lifestyle, and she hopes this can help others find peaceful nights too. Her life since then has become happier, and she has seen much more energy for the day when she wakes up. Helping you to build good habits to sleep better profoundly matters to the author because what you're about to learn is what Callie wished to know many years ago when she was having disturbed nights and low energy in her day-to-day life. It took up to two years to build a good routine that was easy to follow and worked very well. This practical guide is now shared with you all to support you in creating long-lasting habits.

CHAPTER 1: BUILDING LONG-LASTING HABITS

When we define the word habit, we see it is a regular practice of an action or behaviour. Be that exercising, waking up earlier, or taking action. Successful habits, the regular practice of them, lead to a successful and happier life.

Experts say that it takes around 21 days to break or create a habit; this means you can create powerful habits within this short space. However, scientists' studies show that many of us try to build new practices in the wrong way and without following a structure, and after a couple of months, if not weeks, we forget about why we wanted to create this new habit, and we never go back to it. Our mind feels disappointed, and we judge so much our failure that we do not try again. What if we could create a habit and maintain it for a very long time? How proud would we feel about ourselves?

Whenever you build a habit, reflect making it around five essential questions:

- **WHY?** - The core reason for your habit. Ask yourself why you want to create this habit until you know the most profound answer. Why do you want to implement this habit? Why is it important to you? Why is it going to make you happy? Why do you want to be healthier? Why, why, why, get to that reason, so the day you lack motivation, your "why" will be powerful enough to give you the push to keep going.

- **WHAT?** - What is the habit itself, what it involves, what benefits will it bring to your life? If exercising, are you thinking of a particular exercise? Become specific about your habit. If you want to wake up earlier, at what time exactly do you want to wake up? Keep looking for the most particular answers until your response has no space for questions or doubts.

- **HOW?** - How are you going to make this habit happen? Maybe you will wake up earlier by going to sleep earlier, or you are going to exercise more by hiring a personal trainer. And which tools do you need to make sure you are ready to take action?

- **WHEN/WHERE?** - Consider the space. Are you going to train inside or outside? Is it going to be early in the morning or in the afternoon? When are you free? Check the weather to help you with your decision. If it is sleeping, will you sleep somewhere different these days, or will your space be always ready when you decide to sleep? Do you have any reunions at the weekend? Will you have noise around at a particular time? Maybe let your partner know that you will need a quieter environment from 10:30 PM. Space and time are essential for the routine and no interruptions. Think ahead, plan your schedules so you know you will be able to commit to that routine.

- **WHO?** - This is a fundamental question. There are three main questions inside; with who you are going to share your new habit? Who are you going to tell about this habit? And who are you going to learn from so you can keep building this habit? Maybe your friend is ready to exercise more, so you will have a goal together. Perhaps you want to sleep better and earlier, so you will tell your partner that you will practice a good sleeping habit. And you might not know much about how you can keep incorporating new ideas into this new habit, so you can use books or even coaches that will guide you into keeping you focused on your new routine. Inviting others to participate in the same habit will give you a sense of community and belonging. You can feel empathy towards other people's feelings while feeling proud of yourself, too. Telling others about your new habit sets you up with commitment, building self-discipline and determination. You are in continuous development, and you need to fill yourself with the knowledge to keep your habit healthy and long-lasting.

Reward yourself- This is not a question but an action to empower yourself. There is nothing better than rewarding yourself for practicing new habits. This act will reaffirm that you are going through the right path. It will allow you to review what you have achieved and learned, reinforcing the focus on practicing your habit.

As I said before, successful habits lead to a successful and happier life. Like everything, you must have a structure of your habit to build it correctly; this is the only way it will maintain itself. This new structure not only works for sleeping habits. You can use this same structure to build new long-lasting habits in any aspect of your life. You might feel that it has a lot of work on it initially, but it becomes easier over time. Can you imagine building all the healthy habits that you have ever wanted by just following this structure and seeing that it works? Remember, stick to a pace you can follow, do not try to apply five habits at once because those will fail. Just like an architect needs to create one step at a time, you are in charge of making sure that your new habit incorporates successfully in your life.

Now, spend some time identifying all the triggers and obstacles you may have when starting with a new habit. It will help you to get over bad days without going back to old habits. A solid plan, which you will create by answering the above questions, will allow you to quickly get back on track when you skip your new habit. Sometimes you will skip a good habit, and it does not mean you are failing. Think towards your good routine with self-compassion rather than self-judgment. What went wrong? Perhaps you lacked the motivation and realised that your "why" was not strong enough to motivate you. Whatever it was, go back to those questions and find more robust answers, and this will lead you to successful results. Building new habits take patience and consistency. It may be hard if you have never had any good habit in your routine. But if you judge yourself, you will feel less motivated to continue and more encouraged to go back to your old habits. However, when practising self-compassion, you feel love towards yourself, which gives you the strength to see what went wrong so you can correct it instead of feeling guilty about it. Practice self-compassion, and you will have high motivation in life, allow yourself always to want to learn and grow.

"You, as much as anybody in the entire universe, deserve your love and affection"- Buddha.

As far as I have decided to give you the key to building successful habits, I will also release, in the following chapters, sleeping habits that will aid you mentally and physically in your day today. These are seven habits that will improve your sleep quality, basing myself on my experience and applying the five questions mentioned in this first chapter.

I built long-lasting habits because I want a stable life. Do you want to build long-lasting habits? Answer the five questions, create a plan and motivate yourself through your community and self-rewards.

CHAPTER 2: YOUR BEDROOM IS YOUR SAFE PLACE

Your bedroom is a temple. As much as we think that we only sleep in it, we also recharge and create in there. Allow your mind to have a holistic perspective towards your bedroom. Your bedroom is a safe place because it safeguards you when you sleep and welcomes you anytime you are tired. It is a place for creation and a place where creativity expands. There is no other safer place than your bedroom when you set it up correctly. What do I mean by setting up a bedroom correctly? Do you make your bed when you wake up? Are your bedsheets clean? Is your space full of light and tidy? If your bedroom is not clean, you won't feel clean as it is the mirror of yourself. This chapter is about creating a bedroom routine that will make you feel cleaner in the morning and lighter at night.

We spoke in the first chapter about creating a habit. This chapter is about the ritual of creating a safe place for your body to feel that it is allowed to rest deeply. You are reading this to understand in-depth that the "WHERE and WHEN" are essential. And these two questions are connected to your sense of smell and vision.

Let's talk first about what your eyes see. Firstly, once you wake up, the first thing you want to achieve is making your bed. It might sound strange, everyone makes their beds, but

I can only judge myself. Why do you want to make your bed right when you stand up from bed in the morning? Because this small action sets you up for the rest of the day, and it has a much more significant impact once you return home because you find an organised, clean bedroom that invites you to find comfort between your bedsheets and rest. If your bedroom was not clean and tidy, would you feel safe there?

There are other things to consider, such as the lighting of the bedroom or your mattress. Invest some time in observing your bedroom. What do you like? What would you change? Feel your bedroom like your safe place. How can you feel safe? Maybe any time you see your bedsheets you don't like them, so you don't feel comfortable there. Throw them away! Will changing the pillow allow you to have less neck pain? Get a good quality pillow! Invest in what you will prefer for your bedroom to become your temple. Another important aspect of your bedroom is the clutter that you have around. Take some time to remove anything that should not be in your bedroom. Several studies show that untidy bedrooms lead to poor night sleep and anxiety. In Feng-Shui, an ancient oriental practice, decluttering promotes positive energy by harmonising the surrounding environment; hence clutter is stuck energy. Do not underestimate the effect of clutter in your bedroom. The more thoroughly you declutter, the lighter your bedroom will feel. So if you have many clothes in a chair, take that chair away from your bedroom, which will help you not accumulate clothes there. The action of decluttering will make you feel lighter in your body, mind and spirit. Allow movement of energy in your bedroom, conserving what healthy energy is inside only. Take a moment to reflect on what your eyes see, and then keep reading. We are going to learn what our nose senses.

Our body will reject any unpleasant smell from our environment. Where is your laundry? If you have a place to put your dirty laundry and it is out of your bedroom, great! If not, make sure your dirty laundry is covered and far away from your bed, so your nose does not get disturbed by smells. You might also want to start using aromatherapy as a method for bringing a calming sensation to your body. The birthplace of aromatherapy is Ancient Egypt. Can you believe that Ancient Egypt would use essential oils for cosmetics, religion and medicinal purposes 3000 years ago? Khypi, the twenty-three ingredients mixed, was used as a tranquilliser, alleviating anxiety and lightning the pharaoh's dreams. In today's world, we have forgotten about smells that are powerful tools to relax our mind before we sleep and after. You have options such as candles or diffusers that you can use with a few drops of natural essential oils, which will disperse a relaxing smell around your bedroom, maintaining a soothing environment. You can also use these oils by mixing some drops with water and spraying them directly into your pillow. I will list the best essential oils that I recommend you to use:

Lavender oil: it is the most popular oil for relaxation. It promotes relaxation not only in your body but also in your mind. Some studies consider this oil useful in treating anxiety, allergies, depression, insomnia, nausea and even menstrual cramps! This oil is my absolute favourite. When I started using it, I would spray it into my pillow, so I could feel I was in a cosy cloud full of calm when I would smell it.

Ylang Ylang essential oil: Ylang Ylang comes from a tree native to the Philippines and Indonesia. It is famous for its health benefits, such as reducing stress levels and relieving pain and insomnia. A few drops of Ylang Ylang in a diffuser will create a calming and happier sensation in your environment as it is scientifically proven to enhance your serotonin levels, the happiness hormone, and libido!

Frankincense, used in Ancient Egypt, mentioned in the biblical text and given to Jesus as a gift. This oil helps your body reach its ideal temperature for a night of better sleep by promoting relaxation. I recommend using it in the evenings and at any space in the house.

Whatever actions you choose to take from this chapter, such as rearranging the room, start making your bed every morning, or using oils, so your bedroom smells better, remember that one action will lead you to your goal of achieving better sleep. Why? Because you would have had an intention to take care of your temple. Your eyes and your nose are potent senses, and they can make you either have beautiful dreams or nightmares through the night. Energy keeps moving or might be stuck, so do not be shy to explore and re-organise whatever you can feel will improve your night's sleep. Once you think that the "WHERE and WHEN" are set up correctly, you can keep strengthening your habits for a night of better sleep. And do not forget to reward yourself for taking a step into creating a safe place for yourself.

CHAPTER 3: YOU ARE WHAT YOU EAT

Food is the fuel for our body, so it is a crucial aspect of our overall health. In this chapter, we are going to talk about "HOW". How do we make sure we are going to sleep better? How will our diet influence our sleeping? How can I make sure one choice from yesterday will change how I wake up today? Food affects our physical, mental and emotional well-being. A good food diet rich in fruits, vegetables, and whole-grain has been proven to improve optimal brain health, physical health and promotes better sleep. Diets rich in high-sugar, high-carbohydrate and heavily processed foods can influence your rest negatively. Junk food isn't troubling only for our body weight but also for our sleep. Foods containing lots of sugar can cause harm to your blood and your sleeping patterns. Sugar gives our brain a strong signal to be awake, but once that quick fuel, sugar, is finished, our energy levels fall sharply and consume all the energy we had. And this can happen in the morning, afternoon, or evening. It does not matter what time you will eat food that is low in nutrients. They will always give the same effect: first, not having enough food to satisfy your hunger, and secondly, of not giving you enough energy for the rest of the day.

Junk food can make you feel sleepy afterwards, right, but do you feel comfortable once you go to sleep with your stomach full? You feel satisfied as if things are great, but your body is alarmed by the quantity of lousy food it has to get rid of, so you are putting your body to work while you sleep, and so it cannot support you, giving you bad dreams.

Start listing down all of your bad eating habits and try to find healthier alternatives. This action will not just improve your sleep but also your body, mind and spirit. You will be surprised how good healthy food can taste. It is so good that when you try junk food again, you won't like it anymore. Does this mean that if you eat a lot of healthy food at night, this won't happen? Incorrect. You will still keep your body busy with lots of food that needs to get shared between one part of your body or another. Think of your body as a fridge, and the food you put in your mouth is the whole grocery shopping you have done today. If you buy too much, it collapses, you have no more room for it, so you must keep working and re-organising the space for everything to fit inside it. But if you do just a small shopping, or if you see you have enough and can "survive" for a few more hours, you add tranquillity and can concentrate on other things from your life. The body acts the same way. If it has too much going on in the stomach, it might not focus on the most important thing at night: providing a quality of sleep. Instead, the mind will take charge and bring you nightmares about your day, and it will get you heaviness from the food you have eaten. Even the body is going to give signals to the brain to make you feel uncomfortable sleeping!

Once you have found all those small bad habits that contribute to insufficient sleep, replace them with other practices to better sleep. One of them is breakfast. What I am going to say may sound mandatory but, do not skip breakfast! It is the most important meal of the day, and it brings you the energy you need; it makes you less hungry overall. And of course, go for a most fulfilling breakfast! One of the breakfasts that have provided me with the most energy is porridge with nuts and fruits. You can add a teaspoon of honey or cinnamon, make it fun for your eyes, and you will feel the difference. Porridge is excellent as a breakfast because of its filling properties and because it improves your gut movements; it is full of fibre; it will aid you with your bathroom routines. There is a saying that recommends you to eat like a King when you have breakfast because it is the meal you need the most from the other mains. Once you go into your lunch, eat like a prince because you are already half-day away, and your breakfast was healthy enough to fuel you up to the afternoon. Incorporate more greens in your plate, a bit less meat. But even if you are a meat-eater, try to have only the quantity that health professionals recommend.

Did you know that it takes between two and four hours to digest 40g of red meat? Three times the amount of vegetables that digest in 20 minutes. I mean, see the quality of food, how good is it going to be for your body? The body speaks, sometimes the gut complains and makes growling sounds. It is hard for the stomach to digest it, so it is stressed. This stress goes into your body, too, making you feel uncomfortable, bulky, and too full to think clearly. By now, you got the idea. A prince meal is a food portion that satisfies but does not fill you up. That is going to give you fuel instantly and not make you feel sleepy for two hours. You want food that will support your day at the pace that you want.

Once you arrive home, consider eating as if you are on a tight food budget in the evening. Lighter meals in the evening with a two to three hours gap before going to sleep is more than adequate. And this gap is the one that will allow you to have a stomach that will not complain to your mind, and so your body will concentrate on your sleep patterns, making sure that you finally have the right moment of sleep.

You can plan your meals to build a conscious eating habit. This action will improve your gut health and give you a strong immune system. It will also improve your mood, brain health, heart, digestion and especially reward you with a calming sleep sensation. I invite you and encourage you to do some research on the importance to build healthy eating habits. Start with small changes, and they will have a substantial positive impact on your lifestyle.

Now that we spoke about solids, let's talk about liquids! Water is an essential nutrient for the functionality of our body. Some studies have shown that not drinking enough water during the day links to lousy night sleep. During the night, our body goes through a process where we lose liquids by digesting food (imagine how much water we are losing at night if we have to digest a heavy meal!) and breathing and sweating. We must have between 1.5L to 2L of water daily. Water is magical. It alleviates headaches, reduces your stress, hydrates your body, and it prevents heart diseases as well. The best routine you can have with water is to drink one glass of room temperature water once you wake up, before having any other meal, and one glass of water before you sleep. You will see the difference not only in your body but also in your mood. We are mainly water!

If you feel that you are not a water person, but you like tea, you could have a more calming tea in the evening. I do not want to say that tea can be a substitute for water. It cannot. Water purely has the most hydration for the body, while tea does not hydrate the body enough. However, I recommend these two types of teas that have become my best friends for stressful days and disturbed nights. Lavender tea is widely known today for stimulating areas of the brain that supports the boost of your mood and produce calming effects, and it also helps with anxiety and fatigue. Drinking lavender tea at night is ideal if you wish to have a "strong" flavour in your mouth, but still, you want to find peace in your mind. The second one is, of course, chamomile. Chamomile was used in ancient times as a cold remedy and to heal wounds. When

I was a child, we would put the chamomile flowers to boil and then use them to clean our eyes or injuries. Today, people know the calming effect of chamomile tea. It is high in antioxidants that promote relaxation, also easing anxiety and depression. It also has other benefits, such as reducing inflammation and improving the digestive system.

Valerian root has high tranquillity benefits, and you can see the use in pills or other more natural drugs. It is a firm root, and you can find it in its most natural form and make tea with it. This tea can support you if you have insomnia. Because it will be in a raw state, you can benefit from its nutrients better, but control the usage into small quantities as it is a powerful root.

CHAPTER 4: WASH AWAY YOUR WORRIES

When I say to wash your worries away, I mean it.

Our body is mainly water, 60% of water. The ritual of taking a shower is an ancient cleaning practise believed to help balance the body and calming down the nerves. Was your day stressful? Wash your stress away. Have you been worried the whole day about something you have no control of? Wash that worry away. The action of taking a shower always makes you feel positive and fresh. But you want to be clean not only because you will have a long day but also because taking a shower can throw away the negative thoughts that the mind holds during the day. Every day thousands of people with thousands of worries walk through the same streets that you and you collect these worries through your senses: meetings, bad manners from strangers, negative content in social media, negative phone calls, and spilt coffee and so on.

You might wake up and have a shower before going on with your day. That is great because that shower set you up for a new day. You used this shower as a tool to awaken yourself, and psychologically your mind took the signal of being ready. A whole day passes by, and you arrive home feeling tired or upset about something. The mind is waiting for the same signal that you give in the morning to know that you are transitioning from work mode into resting mode. So, the best tool is then the shower. You told your mind that you arrived at the end of your day, and you are ready to jump into bed to rest. This evening shower is the closure of your daily routine, and it leaves behind everything that happened during the day. This ritual is repeated every day, like the sunrise and the sunset.

Most people would typically want to have only a warm shower in the evening because it will relax them completely. In this chapter, I intend to talk you through the benefit of using both cold and hot water to maintain that relaxation moment through the night by benefiting your body system into better health.

On the one hand, hot baths stimulate a calming and relaxing sensation. These feelings send signals to our brain, saying that "it's time to sleep". Paradoxically, TV and movies have also contributed to this connection of hot water and bedtime connection, reassuring us that we would not feel rested if we do not have a hot bath. However, in this present time where worries, anxieties and stress from the city overtakes our lives, things become more complicated, we do not have time for hot baths every day, and our bills would be costly at the end of the month. That is why then we take hot showers, and we simulate the same effect. On this occasion, however, I want to recommend to you the use of cold water right at the end of your hot shower.

There is this misconception that if you are going to shower, you must have only a cold-water shower. But not even the bravest ones would do this every day of their lives. What you might only need is between 15 and 30 seconds of cold water in your body. You want to create an "alarm" system for your body that will awaken your cells and stimulate your blood circulation. Why? Because this blood circulation will calm your body system down, hence you will feel relaxed. The whole purpose is to sleep, and I know it may sound strange to say that your body will feel awake. But this does not last the entire night. It actually might last around 5 minutes. After that, your body feels lighter, and the system is reset to zero, ready to be put to sleep.

Have you ever noticed how you start feeling hot too quickly once you go between your bedsheets and are not comfortable anymore, wishing that you had some little cold air around to feel cosy and wrapped again? Your body can be that cold air. You will feel wrapped in something warm, comfortable, hugging you and inviting you to sleep better.

Other benefits of a cold shower are acting as stress relief; this is because the body is only concentrating on the present moment, not having time to create troubles in mind. It also strengthens the immune system by increasing the number of white cells (our defence cells) in our bodies. Even if it is winter, this habit will boost your defences and protect you against diseases.

Your skin will glow up because cold water improves blood circulation; your skin will be more active at receiving oxygen. When the legs are tired, cold water is magical at reducing inflammation and preventing varicose veins from appearing.

Psychologically, introducing cold showers into your daily routine will empower your self-discipline. You will be building a strong mind to last, even if it is thirty seconds, in cold water. Of course, this habit may take some practice, determination, sometimes more than courage, but ask yourself why you want to do this—having a thirty seconds cold shower is a habit that reinforces your sleep pattern and your immune system. You have the choice of not trying it because you don't like cold water, or you have the option of trying it once, at least once and check how you feel afterwards.

If you decide to follow this habit, follow the six questions from chapter 1. Find a powerful "WHY" that will remind you why you choose ten seconds of cold water every day. Find a way of making it work for you. Maybe thirty seconds is too much for you, and 15 seconds are enough. Think about the tools you need, such as your pyjama on hand, or maybe you only want to feel some cold in your body, so you are OK in a towel. If you have office hours, plan when you know you will have to shower, so you commit to your schedule. Maybe you want to do it every other day. That is fine as well as long as you reflect on your new habit and use the tools from chapter one to succeed. Notice the change in your skin, the difference in your mood, the change in your sleep. Tell someone that you will do it for some time to test it out and commit to it for a certain period. Invite your friends, your partner, and your parents to test it out!

If you doubt it at some point, think again about why you decided to do this. If you decide that this is not for you, do not give up yet. When you try it for some time is when you have a word to say. Find your most profound reason and sleep well.

CHAPTER 5: TIME TO DISCONNECT

We believe in disconnecting from real life once we go into our electronic devices. We also think that maybe by turning on the TV we will fall asleep. But how do our eyes feel once we wake up? Our body and cells have an automated biological clock. It works around a 24-hour sleep-wake cycle. This cycle works together with two hormones in our body: cortisol and melatonin. When we wake up, our cortisol levels rise, so we start feeling awake and alert. And when the night arrives, our body produces melatonin, and hence we feel sleepy. Our cells also have a biological clock, and we are entirely different every day. We have billions of cells, and every six months, we have changed all the cells of our body!

In this chapter, time to disconnect; is not related to disconnecting yourself. It is allowing you to disconnect from whichever device you use at night. Now that we have modern technology, we can bring all the world through an electronic device to bed. However, electronic devices such as cell phones, television, tablets, etc., emit a blue light which delays the natural production of melatonin, the hormone that makes us feel sleepy, and encourages this awake feeling instead. Don't you wonder why you feel exhausted in the morning if you have been using an electronic device too long at night? Even if we fall asleep after 2 hours of watching TV, the body will remain unconsciously awake, and we will wake up most likely tired the following day. You can say that this is your habit, and you might not fall asleep if you don't have the TV on or check any social media. But which kind of a habit is that? Is it empowering you and encouraging your body to fall asleep? Or is it giving you anxiety and promoting for you to be awake more hours? We are going to work on REPLACING this bad habit with a new healthy before-bed habit.

Using chapter one as guidance, list down the time you spend in the evening using electronic devices and set yourself a time to stop. Let's say you want to go to bed at 10:30 PM because you need to wake up at 6:30 AM. You want to allow your body to stop receiving that blue light from your electronic devices so your melatonin can kick in. You can feel that it's time to sleep, so I recommend you leave your phone in a little box where you know it's safe but not to be touched anymore until the next day, half an hour before 10:30 PM. Remember that once you go to bed, it will take you another 30 min to find comfortable and fall asleep, so your actual sleep time will be approximately 11 PM. If you still think that leaving the phone somewhere won't work and you will be tempted to take it, then you can turn it off until the next day. When you turn your phone off, you also disconnect from it. It's a switch off the bottom, not only for the screen but also for yourself. The second option is to turn off the notifications or switch on aeroplane mode, so you know that you won't receive notifications distracting you from your main goal: having eight hours of sleep. To turn the phone off and leave it in another room is another radical option if you know you will be cheating and taking your phone straight away after 10min because you forgot to write a message that can wait for tomorrow.

When we switch off our devices, we unconsciously allow our mind to have the space to rest and concentrate only on the present act of sleeping. You tell your mind that it is correct to focus on falling asleep because your phone is also "sleeping". After this, you want to make sure that you replace your phone at night with another habit. Firstly, some of the tricks that work is having a small notebook or post-it notes to write positive things that happened in your day. It will put you in the present moment and will inspire you to feel positive about yourself. You can also replace your phone by introducing a paper book for your night routine. You do not need to be reading for two hours. Even 10 minutes can do the job. Sometimes the mind only wants to be distracted because it is not good at keeping itself at ease. Have you realised by now how I treat your mind as another entity apart from yourself? You should try this too. Your mind separates from your body entirely, and most of the time, the mind wins control over the body. You must start controlling your mind's thoughts so you can gain control back of it so that if the mind says, "let's take the phone and be awake for two more hours", you can answer, "instead, I would like to read a book while I have a cup of tea and then sleep eight hours". The mind will try sabotaging you, but you will gain control over yourself only by listening to it and answering with confidence. You can strengthen this at night by introducing guided meditations that will allow you to be in the present.

So why do you want to disconnect from devices before going to sleep? And why do you want to sleep better? Get to that powerful "WHY", discover the healthy habit. The mind will try to control you, but you are the real owner of your life. Some days it might be hard, some others, you won't be bothered, but it is in those moments where you will feel proud of yourself for not falling into temptation. If you fail, do not give up and learn a new method. You will master your night habits, and you will master your life!

CHAPTER 6: 10 MINUTES IN ACTION

By now, we all know the benefits of exercising. And that is why I decide to mention it in this book. Exercise is not only to lose weight; it is also to help you sleep. How? Make sure you utilise a good amount of energy throughout the day, so you arrive home with not enough physical strength to be awake until 2 AM. Would you like to fall asleep faster at night? You need as little as 10 minutes of exercise to improve the quality of your sleep. Ten minutes of walking or 10 minutes of scrolling down in social media? This chapter is about you, about you and your relationship with time. Time can be as short as you want it to be, as dull as you want it to be, and as powerful as you want it to be.

You have in your power time and yourself. You can choose how you want to be active and how long you want your body to be involved in the movement. Only 10 minutes is what you need, but you can always be active for more time. The more time you spend doing any activity that involves your body's movement, the better you will feel, the more stress you will release, and the more energy you will spend so you will go to sleep faster. Do not misinterpret me, though; this does not mean that you should start having a 1-hour exercise every day for then failing one week after, no. This chapter is for you to understand how time is your friend and how to be "active" does not mean going to the gym but making your legs and arms move more. Let's check different types of not-so-good-habits.

Let's say that you spend seven hours in front of a computer Monday to Friday and that you have one hour break. In your break, you sit down and eat. Eating will take more and less twenty minutes. You still have another forty minutes to spare, so you go to your phone and scroll down on social media and chat with friends. Once you finish your break, you go back to your office and continue with your work. After work, you arrive home, put on comfortable clothes, and lay on the sofa and watch anything on the TV. Finally, it is time to sleep, you still feel awake, and your body is not comfortable. You start wondering why you are not tired if the day was long, you worked, you were stressed, you did so much at work, and still, you cannot sleep. But actually, did your body do much at work? No. Your body barely moved!

Another approach is investing 10 minutes to ensure that your body moves. So, if you know that you won't move at all while you are in the office, you still have 30 minutes spare from your break where you can stand up and go outside, maybe you can call a friend for 10 minutes while you surround the building instead of being sat waiting for time to pass by through social media. You want to make sure you allow your body to feel useful. Your body also asks for some work, just like your mind does. Otherwise, it won't let you sleep through the night.

If you feel that those 30 minutes break are not for you to move, set an activity outside. Have a schedule also for that specific time, just as if it was part of work. You can also check how long it would take you to go to work walking so you can move before going to work. Thirty minutes walking is perfectly achievable, it will also give you time to listen to a podcast while you go to work and set you up in an excellent mood, and you will be saving money too!

Did you know that exercise reduces the risk of developing insomnia and sleep apnea? No pills will help you more than exercising in the morning or evening. Choose a time, build a habit, go back to chapter one and check the tools you need. Maybe you want to create every day 10 minutes' walk habit. Perhaps you want to start walking from work to home three times per week. Stretching also counts as an activity, so why not trying some ten minutes of stretching yoga. All activities will increase the duration of your sleep. If you wake up many times at night, the body tells you that it has stopped for so long that it needs to move. It wants to move! And once you move for ten minutes, you will feel great, boosted with energy in the day.

You can choose when you want to practise this ten-minutes body movement. If you feel that you are more active in the morning, maybe you want to do a bit more intense exercise to arrive at the end of the day ready to go to bed and fall asleep.

On the other hand, if you feel that evening is when you want to move after a long day, some relaxing movements such as yoga or stretching will help you bring the body back to a more relaxed state. Everyone is different; explore your options. You are ready to start!

CHAPTER 7: TRAVEL TO COMFORT

When I hear the word "travelling", my heart jumps with emotion because I know travelling is exciting. It means that I am going to explore and that I am going to learn different things. But I also know that I must prepare myself. I want things to go right. What if it rains? What if the place has no potable water? I also apply the word travelling when I go to work, so I feel excited that even if I do not go out of the country, I will travel somewhere, and I will enjoy the ride. Even for this, I prepare myself. I must check the time I start and finish, my uniform, my lunch, travel card, the weather! I also travel back from anywhere to my home, my comfort zone. At home, I can be myself. I am safe. This chapter is about you, about me, and travelling.

This habit is about setting up a time to go to sleep every night. From the set time, go to bed thirty minutes before to allow your body and mind to get comfortable. From the moment you stand up from your living room sofa, and you move into your bed. The bed is the vehicle that will transport you on a journey of 8 hours so you can reset yourself, so you can keep travelling each day of your life. There are tools that you need: your mind must be present. Have you noticed how much your mind starts to think once you go to bed? Some studies show that the mind is more creative at night time; hence it awakens and starts exploring different scenarios from past weeks, or sometimes years! This overthinking can lead us to feel guilt, sometimes anger or frustration.

Has anyone told you, ever, that the best way to go to sleep is to feel your heart light? To hear about a light heart before going to sleep was life-changing for me. I kept listening to it once and twice, and then a third time in different countries. I asked a wise man how I could sleep better, and he said, "Once you go to sleep, forgive and forget. Forgive the person that caused the pain and forget the pain that caused on you". In the beginning, I could not understand, but I could see peace in his eyes. He said, "It is important to forgive others, do not hold your heart full of pain, or it won't let you sleep at night". And he was right. A stranger in the middle of Egypt's bazaar was teaching me how I could sleep better. Of course, then I kept researching until I understood that forgiving is also healing. You heal your wounds, the marks you have in your heart or mind, forgive what hurts in your day and the person who wanted to cause that harm because they are lost souls that do not have yet found peace. You forgive and heal those wounds so you can sleep peacefully at night. Why do you think the baby's sleep so well? They do not hold themselves frustrated. They are happy beings, they love sleeping, and they sleep peacefully. Have a baby mind!

The other practice is gratitude, saying thank you to your partner for being there when you need it or showing love every day through small acts. Gratitude can also be towards yourself, thank yourself for taking steps into a better habit, thank yourself for moving more, and eating better. Practising gratitude allows you to be present. It also allows you to experience accomplishment and happiness, stopping your mind from feeling negativity. It might sound like going out of the purpose of sleeping well, but the cause of most of our sleeping problems are the negative feelings our mind creates at night, the overwhelming and almost uncontrollable overthinking. That is why you want to make sure that you bring your mind to the present moment and a happier state: gratitude and forgiveness.

Forgive the one that hurt, and be thankful to the one that made you smile, where your thoughts can be light, and your heart can be content, so your body can relax and take that journey of complete relaxation. And just as if you were travelling to another place, how would your trip be better? With a backpack full of heavy things that you do not necessarily need or with a light bag with only practical things? Take the habit of thinking about sleeping as if it was a trip that you take every day within yourself. Some days the journey may be challenging. Ask yourself what it is making your trip harder. This travelling considers where you are going, how you will travel, why you will travel, and who you will travel with. Your mind will try to obstruct your journey to achieve a long-lasting habit. Feel compassion for your mind whenever you feel resistance, and ask yourself again why you decided to take on this journey. This chapter is a deeper level of consciousness. It is a level of practical guidance for the energy that you have within yourself. This chapter involves your feelings being accountable for your sleeping and yourself as the guide to teach you again everything you knew and did not realise by allowing emotions to come and go while you feel compassion. This journey reassures you that you are taking steps towards better health. Improving your sleep quality will be successful from a conscious place of forgiveness, gratitude, and self-love.

CHAPTER 8: YOGA NIDRA MEDITATION

This chapter is an exercise for your body and mind. You only need a voice recorder for this habit, as I will provide you with the guided meditation you can use. This chapter is about the "WHO". Who are you going to share this reflection with so it will improve their sleep quality? Who are you going to be practising this guided meditation with? What community will surround you and explain to you about their personal experiences when they practised this meditation? This habit is built. There won't be a need to change and think about which meditation you want to listen to, it can always be the same, and it will always give you powerful results. This meditation frees you from worries, and it lets you, peacefully, find your path to sleep.

In this chapter, I want to talk briefly about "Yoga Nidra". Yoga Nidra is an ancient technique from India that brings you to a going-to-sleep" stage in your consciousness, and it intends for you to relax all parts of your body through guided meditation. This meditation practice invites you to dive into a deep relaxation mood by focusing your attention on one part of the body mentioned and allowing it to relax. For the best result, I encourage you to record yourself and play it back. You can also ask someone else to record it for you if you feel that your voice will distract you instead of relaxing. I invite you to explore how your body becomes deeply relaxed, one part at a time.

This practice must be recorded slowly, with a calming voice, mentioning every word. Allow time between one sentence and another. There is an example with the word "pause", where you should be allowing some pause before you mention the next body part. Once you are ready, have your body laying down (Shavasana position in yoga), feet separated apart from each other and hands on each side of the body.

"Breath normally (pause)

Left hand (pause)

The thumb of your left-hand, (pause) RELAX

2nd finger, RELAX

3rd finger, RELAX

4th finger, RELAX

5th finger, RELAX

All five fingers of your left hand RELAX.

Left palm, RELAX

Left wrist, RELAX

Left lower-arm up to the elbow, RELAX

The left upper-arm, from shoulder to the elbow, RELAX

Left shoulder, RELAX

All left arm, RELAX

Right-hand thumb, RELAX

2nd finger, RELAX

3rd finger, RELAX

4th finger, RELAX

5th finger, RELAX

All five fingers from your right hand, RELAX.

Right palm, RELAX

Right wrist, RELAX

Right lower-arm up to the elbow, RELAX

The right upper arm, shoulder to the elbow, RELAX

Right shoulder, RELAX

All right arm, RELAX

Left foot big toe, RELAX

2nd toe, RELAX

3rd toe, RELAX

4th toe, RELAX

 5th toe, RELAX

All five toes of your left foot, RELAX

Left Foot, RELAX

Left ankle, RELAX

Left lower-leg up to the knee, RELAX

Left knee, RELAX

Left thigh, RELAX

Left hip, RELAX

All left leg, RELAX

Breath normally

Right leg, right foot

Right big toe, RELAX

2nd toe, RELAX

3rd toe, RELAX

4th toe, RELAX

5th toe, RELAX

All five toes of your right foot, RELAX

Right foot, RELAX

Right ankle, RELAX

Right lower-leg up to the knee, RELAX

Right knee, RELAX

Right thigh, RELAX

Right hip, RELAX

All right leg, RELAX

All left leg, RELAX

All right arm, RELAX

All left arm, RELAX

Walst, RELAX

Breath normally

Stomach, RELAX

Chest, RELAX

Left collarbone, RELAX

Right collarbone, RELAX

Upper-back, RELAX

Lower-back, RELAX

Top of the head now

Forehead, RELAX

Right eyebrow, RELAX

Left eyebrow, RELAX

Right eyelid, RELAX

Left eyelid, RELAX

Right eyeball, RELAX

Left eyeball, RELAX

Right nostril, RELAX

Left nostril, RELAX

All nose, RELAX

Upper-lip, RELAX

Lower-lip, RELAX

Tongue in your mouth, RELAX

Lower-jaw, RELAX

Upper-jaw, RELAX

Right cheek, RELAX

Left cheek, RELAX

Right ear, RELAX

Left ear, RELAX

Back of your neck, RELAX

Front of your neck, RELAX

All head, RELAX

All upper-body, RELAX

All lower-body, RELAX

All body, RELAX

Continue breathing normally

You are relaxed. Your body is relaxed,

Breath normally

Listen to the sounds inside the room,

Listen to the sounds outside this room,

Your body is relaxed

At peace, deep relaxation

Breath normally,

Ohmmmmmmmmmm,

Ohmmmmmmmmmm,

Ohmmmmmmmmmm

After this meditation, you will feel the sense of floating, almost as if your body left you: no aches, only you and the calming sensation of floating in clouds. Once you are in bed, this will be great for you to fall asleep instantly. Remember to go back to the present moment by opening your eyes slowly, with no rush, and make tiny moves in each part of your body until you become present completely. Enjoy the journey to a restful night's sleep.

CONCLUSION

I hope this book gave you the tools to build long-lasting habits for a more successful life. Remember to apply the key takeaway of each chapter: Optimise your bedroom environment, maintain a healthy diet, and take showers that will clean your body and mind. Minimise blue light before bedtime, let your body move, commit to a sleep schedule and practise guided meditation. Improving your sleep quality will be successful from a conscious place of forgiveness, gratitude, and self-love. These practices will improve the quality of your sleep and the quality of your life.

PLEASE, LEAVE A REVIEW IF YOU ENJOYED THIS BOOK!

RESOURCES

11 Steps to Creating the Perfect Bedroom for Sleep.
https://www.goodhousekeeping.com/health/wellness/advice/a25468/bedroom-sleep-tips/

Best Essential Oils for Sleep **(Sanchita Sen ed., Vol. 1).**
https://amerisleep.com/blog/best-essential-oils-for-sleep/

Decluttering as spiritual practice.
https://magnoliaswest.com/decluttering-as-spiritual-practice/

We are what we eat.
https://brainfitresorts.com/we-are-what-we-eat/*Diet & Sleep:*

Relationship Between Nutrition & Sleep.
https://www.sleepscore.com/eat-well-sleep-well-how-diet-affects-your-sleep/

Benefits of cold showers.
https://www.wimhofmethod.com/benefits-of-cold-showers

How Electronics Affect Sleep.
https://www.sleepfoundation.org/how-sleep-works/how-electronics-affect-sleep